PROBIOTIC DIETING

THE MIRACLE OF PROBIOTICS IN HEALING YOUR GUT, TRIMMING BELLY FAT AND WEIGHT LOSS

I0407857

BY SMART READS

Free Audiobook

As a thank you for being a Smart Reader you can choose
2 FREE audiobooks from audible.com.
Simply sign up for free by visiting
www.audibletrial.com/Travis to get your books.

Visit:
www.smartreads.co/freebooks
to receive Smart Reads books for FREE

Check us out on Instagram:
www.instagram.com/smart_readers
@smart_readers

ABOUT SMARTREADS

Choose Smart Reads and get smart every time. Smart Reads sorts through all the best content and condenses the most helpful information into easily digestible chunks.

We design our books to be short, easy to read and highly informative. Leaving you with maximum understanding in the least amount of time.

Smart Reads aims to accelerate the spread of quality information so we've taken the copyright off everything we publish and donate our material directly to the public domain. You can read our uncopyright below.

We believe in paying it forward and donate 5% of our net sales to Pencils of Promise to build schools, train teachers and support child education.

To limit our footprint and restore forests around the globe we are planting a tree for every 10 hardcover books we sell.

Thanks for choosing Smart Reads and helping us help the planet.

Sincerely,

Travis & the Smart Reads Team

TABLE OF CONTENTS

INTRODUCTION

Have you ever been interested in finding out what probiotics are and how they can boost your digestive system and general health? If so, then this is the book for you. In this book, you will discover the ways science is unraveling the mysteries of maintaining a healthy digestive system so that you can lose weight, trim belly fat, and enjoy your life. The majority of people carry a bit of flab around their belly, but with probiotics, this will no longer be a problem for you. You will be able to shed weight quickly and in a healthy simple way. Let's get going!

CHAPTER 1: DEMYSTIFYING PROBIOTICS

It is hard to believe, much less accept, that someone would deliberately add billions of bacteria to their food every day just to stay healthy. We all know bacteria as disease causing organisms. However, more and more studies are being released showing that particular ailments are treatable and preventable through consumption of food and supplements that contain live bacteria.

The majority of the Northern European diet and culture consists of consumption of beneficial bacteria. A lot of people consume fermented food items that contain bacteria. Two great examples of this are sauerkraut and yoghurt. Japanese culture and Asian culture, in general, provide beverages filled with probiotic.

In Northern America, however, people haven't opened up to consuming probiotic foods, though this has been changing gradually over the last couple of years. Today, there is widespread promotion of diverse probiotic diets.

Understanding What Probiotics Are
Probiotics can be defined as live microorganisms that provide humans and animals with health benefits. There are a number of products currently in the market that incorporate probiotic supplements and foods.

While it is true that microorganisms are usually thought of as dangerous "germs" by most people, there are specific types that actually enable the body to function better. Our digestive systems naturally contain bacteria whose role is to help us digest food, manufacture vitamins, and kill the microorganisms that make us sick. In reality, our bodies contain millions of different microorganisms, with science confirming that the ratio of microorganisms to body cells is 10 to 1. The live microorganisms contained in probiotic food function just as those occurring naturally in the body.

The Discovery of Probiotics

The first person to conceptualize probiotics was the Russian zoologist and microbiologist Ilya Metchnikoff. The term "probiotics" was not being used at the time, but he came up with a theory that particular microorganisms would benefit a person's health if they were added to the diet. Metchnikoff won the Nobel Prize for Physiology in 1908 for his discovery of probiotics, and his fame lives on to this day.

As more research was conducted into the work of Metchnikoff. Scientists coined the term "probiotics" from the Latin term "pro" (for) and the Greek term "biotikos" (fit life). The word probiotics therefore means "for life." In fact, it wasn't until 1965 that the term probiotics was used by two scientists, R.H. Stillwell and D.M. Lilly. They used the term to describe the manner in which a microorganism produced certain secretions to spur the growth of other microbes. This was exactly contrary to how antibiotics worked.

The first person to use the term probiotics to refer to food and supplements containing microorganisms and substances that have the ability to directly influence the balance of digestive microbes in mammals was R.B. Parker. This occurred in 1974, but 15 years later, Roy Fuller, a gut microecology scientist, refined Parker's definition of probiotics. Fuller defined probiotics not as "substances" but "live microbial feed supplements." This was later to be accepted as the modern and official definition of what probiotics is - focusing on their capacity to stay stable and offer healthy benefits to a person.

Probiotics vs. Prebiotics vs. Synbiotics

The three terms above are normally confused as meaning the same thing. However, they are quite distinct. Prebiotics refer to dietary components that support the growth of beneficial bacteria. Synbiotics refer to products that are a combination of probiotics and prebiotics.

Fast Fact: Are you aware that makeup and skin creams contain probiotics?

Probiotic Microbes

There are many different bacteria and microorganisms in probiotics. The two major groups are Lactobacilli and Bifidobacteria. The other forms of bacteria used to manufacture commercial probiotics all fall under these two categories.

Lactobacilli (plural for Lactobacillus) are a group of 180 different species of bacteria, considered to be beneficial to human health. They naturally occur in the digestive, urinary, and genital systems of human beings, and don't cause any diseases.

Bifidobacteria (plural for Bifidobacterium) are bacteria that naturally occur in mammals, specifically in the gastrointestinal tract, genitals, and mouth. They tend to live in the intestines of human beings.

The Status of Probiotics Locally and Internationally

The World Health Organization (WHO) defined probiotics in 2001 as living microorganisms that offer humans health benefits if consumed in sufficient quantities. The United Nation's Food and Agriculture Organization (FAO) and WHO came together in 2002 to develop guidelines for evaluating dietary probiotics. The working group recommended that any health claims made should be validated and assessed. In 2010, academic scientists and industry experts joined the global effort.

Due to increased efforts worldwide to confirm the health benefits claims, there was a major increase in the production and use of probiotics. Asia and Europe were quick to accept it, but America still lagged behind. From 2007 to 2012, the number of adult Americans using probiotics had quadrupled compared to the previous 10 years. Probiotics are currently the most popular diet supplement in America after minerals and vitamins.

In a survey conducted by the National Health Interview Survey (NHIS) in 2012, it was discovered that about 1.6% of American adults and o.5% of children aged between 4 and 17 make use of probiotics on a daily basis. These figures are increasing every year. The value of the probiotics industry as of 2015 was estimated at $2.187 billion, and this is projected to rise to $3.314 billion by 2020. This is a growth rate of 7.6% every year. As the market grows steadily and people learn more about the health benefits of probiotics, its acceptance increases. This has also led to the development of probiotics diets.

CHAPTER 2: UNDERSTANDING THE PROBIOTICS DIET

Our bodies contain about 100 trillion bacteria, both on and inside us. All these bacteria together form what is known as the microbiome, with the biggest collection living inside the human digestive system. These bacteria are referred to as gut flora. Researchers have discovered that having a larger and more diverse microbiome is better for health. It is believed that having friendly bacteria inside the gut is a key aspect of good health.

The problem is that the majority of people have embraced a lifestyle that consists of poor eating habits, thus resulting in depletion of the natural supply of beneficial microorganisms found in gut flora. This poor diet consists of excessive quantities of refined sugars, artificial sweeteners, simple carbs, processed foods, and antibiotics. This kind of diet results in the depletion of the good bacteria found in the gut, and according to recent studies conducted by prominent researchers, the ultimate outcome is inability to maintain or lose weight.

If the gut flora of the human digestive system isn't as diverse as it should be, the body will start to absorb more calories from the food consumed. Regardless of the quantity of food eaten, the person will still continue to gain weight. Furthermore, these microorganisms also affect the hormones that are supposed to regulate one's appetite, for example, leptin and ghrelin.

Apart from helping in weight loss, there are other benefits of the gut having a large quantity of beneficial bacteria. These include good skin, improved emotional state, and an enhanced immune system. People who have incorporated probiotics into their diet have experienced loss of weight and an increase in energy. Other side effects include a reduction in food cravings, mouth ulcers, acne, asthma, and heartburn. Women tend to experience fewer instances of the symptoms of menopause. For people who hate calorie counting or do not want to starve themselves in the name of dieting, a probiotics diet is the answer.

Components of a Probiotics Diet
A probiotics diet is built around following these three components:

•Consuming beneficial bacteria
•Adding beneficial bacteria to different food items
•Combining beneficial bacteria and nutritional supplements

Keeping the body healthy requires one to avoid consuming lifeless, sterilized food. Instead, the diet should primarily consist of traditional, fermented foods that provide adequate probiotics. These types of foods enable easy and safe digestion of raw vegetables and dairy products. They reduce the damage caused by dangerous chemicals and metals found in the environment.

Another benefit is that they aid the body in eliminating toxins and maintain a holistic wellbeing. Every human body is unique, with each having its own number and combination of microorganisms. This microbiome is sustained through a probiotics diet filled with fermented foods, which is much better than consuming probiotics supplements. Consuming a probiotics diet is the best way to reconstruct and restore digestive and immune systems.

Probiotics Dietary Guide
Described below is the most basic probiotics diet that will help guide you through the many variations that exist.

Food Items to Temporarily Abstain From:

Beans
For people who are vegetarians, beans are an excellent protein source. To those who are not vegetarians, beans are to be avoided because they contain lectins, a substance that is known to irritate the stomach lining. Beans can also cause the microorganisms' levels in some people's guts to be unbalanced.

Grains
People on the diet should stay away from grains like rice, oats, and quinoa. This will enable them to consume more fruits and vegetables, thus promoting the growth of healthy bacteria. The gluten content in wheat and rye can also lead to stomach irritation, so these grains should also be avoided by dieters.

Dairy
Cheese and milk should be avoided for a brief time period, and are only to be brought back into the diet later.

Artificial and Natural Sweeteners
The sugar found in fruits can be consumed, but all artificial sweeteners and refined sugars must be avoided. This is because they have the ability to mess up the equilibrium of bacteria in the gut.

Caffeine
The problem with caffeine is that it raises stress hormones and increases the sugar levels in the bloodstream, thus negatively affecting the microbiome. Abstaining from caffeine can be very difficult for those who love drinking coffee daily. The best thing to do to avoid the headaches resulting from caffeine withdrawal is to reduce coffee intake slowly over a two week period prior to starting the

probiotics diet. Great and healthier alternatives include herbal teas or hot water containing ginger and sliced lemon.

Alcohol
The first 4 weeks of the probiotics diet requires total avoidance of all types of alcohol. Alcohol is known to destroy the intestinal mucus that is supposed to protect the body from inflammation and infection. It also interferes with the balance of bacteria, thus resulting in excessive levels of the bad kind of bacteria. If it is too difficult to quit alcohol, it is recommended that the individual drink fizzy water that contains a bit of lime or lemon juice. This too can be an enjoyable drink!

The Initial Two-Week Meal Guide
For anyone planning to start a probiotics diet and lifestyle, the initial two weeks require exclusive consumption of fruits and vegetables, with proteins the only exception. The list of food items is as follows:

•Protein
Eating a small amount of protein daily with every meal can aid in the repair of the intestinal lining. Processed meats like deli meats and cold cuts are to be avoided, but organic meats such as skinless chicken, lean pork and beef, and fish are allowed. Eggs, seeds, and nuts are also good protein choices.

•Vegetables
Vegetables are rich in plant fibers and chemicals, which provide the perfect breeding ground for beneficial bacteria. They help to promote a digestive system that is healthy. For these first two weeks, there should be consumption of a daily minimum of five cups of vegetables. The vegetables can be combined with two cups of fruit. A recommended appetizer for meals is salad comprising bitter leaves and grapefruit

juice, vinegar or lemon. Radicchio, chicory, and endive are bitter leaves that help trigger the production of digestive enzymes. The vinegar, lemon and grapefruit increase the potency of the enzymes, thus helping in the release of stomach acids which further digest food.

•Fruits
Two cups of fruit daily is the recommended amount for a probiotics diet. Blueberries, peaches, kiwis, melons, clementines, bananas, papayas, pears, oranges, and watermelons are considered the best fruits for this diet.

•Non-Dairy Food
When preparing sauces and salad dressings, only coconut or virgin olive oil should be used. They are rich in plant chemicals known as polyphenols, which are known to promote growth of beneficial stomach bacteria. Olive and coconut oils are regarded as healthy fats. However, fats in general, and foods with high fat content specifically, tend to promote growth of bad stomach bacteria. Therefore, coconut and olive oils are to be consumed in moderation.

The Intermediate Two Week Meal Guide
In the third and fourth week of the probiotics diet, vegetarians can go ahead and consume beans in case they were not doing so during the initial two weeks. For non-vegetarians, however, the diet remains exactly the same as for the initial two weeks. It is also now possible to add prebiotic foods to the probiotics diet. Dairy should still be avoided, though fermented cheese may be consumed daily in small portions.

•Probiotics
A single serving of foods rich in probiotics should be eaten every day. Examples of such foods are provided in the final

chapter. When probiotics are introduced into the body, they replenish the good kind of bacteria in the gut, thus helping the individual lose weight and keep it off. On the other hand, it is important that the person opts for fresh, organic, and whole probiotics sources. Pills and dietary supplements are not recommended, and they also tend to be more expensive.

•**Prebiotics**

The list below includes the vegetables and fruits that provide the perfect nourishment to good bacteria:

•Leeks
•Bananas
•Apples
•Onions
•Artichokes
•Pak choi
•Asparagus
•Fennel
•Potatoes (to be served cold)

The foods above can be enjoyed at anytime during the day. In case there is any food in the list above that isn't part of one's regular diet, it should be introduced gradually to prevent gas and bloating.

Maintaining the Diet from the 5th Week Onwards
Once an individual has been on the diet for over four weeks, they can start to add beans and grains into their diet, though only in tiny portions daily. The way the body responds to reintroduction of these foods should be monitored. In case of any negative side effects, for example, mood swings, loss of appetite, pain, or change in the texture of the skin, the serving sizes should be reduced. If symptoms persist, the food item should be totally avoided. The same procedure

should be followed with dairy, caffeine, and alcohol – gradual reintroduction, close monitoring of body responses, and avoidance in case of adverse side effects.

Fast fact: Did you know that the recommended serving of protein for an adult of average size is between 45 to 56 grams daily?

There are a number of lifestyle adjustments that must be made to enable the good bacteria to continue growing in the gut:

1. Probiotics should be consumed daily, combined with a low-fat diet but rich in fiber.

2. Meals should be eaten at definite times of the day. For instance, breakfast at 7 in the morning, lunch at noon, and supper at 6 in the evening. Staying consistent with meal times daily prevents the body from absorbing excess calories and supports the growth of a wider variety of bacteria in the gut.

3. Food should be chewed slowly and in a relaxed manner. This promotes the healing of stomach lining cells, aids in the absorption of nutrients, and stimulates release of digestive acids and enzymes.

4. Ensure that the foods consumed in every meal are wide in variety. The proteins and fruits/vegetables should be put together in diverse combinations. Maintaining variety will prevent boredom while dieting, which is one factor that makes most people regain the weight that had been lost.

A probiotics diet benefits more than just the body's digestive system. Every other body function also enjoys the benefits since it is an interconnected system that must always maintain some sort of balance. A probiotics diet merely emphasizes the fact that a strong digestive system is the first step to total wellness.

CHAPTER 3: BENEFITS OF A PROBIOTICS DIET

There are innumerable health benefits to having the correct number and type of bacteria living in the gut. The main ones include weight loss, better digestion, better skin, and stronger immunity.

How Probiotics Affect the Body
First of all, it is absolutely necessary for a person to have microorganisms in their digestive system. There are about a thousand different species of microorganisms in the gut, including bacteria, viruses, and yeasts. Bacteria are the majority, with most of them living in the colon (large intestine). There are different metabolic functions that take place among the gut flora, and this actually resembles the workings of a body organ. For this reason, some scientists decided to name the large grouping of gut microorganisms "the forgotten organ."

Gut flora is very important for a person's health. It manufactures vitamins such as vitamin K and B. Gut flora provides nourishment for the good bacteria in the stomach by turning dietary fibers into butyrate, propionate, and acetate. These are examples of fatty acids that are absorbed by the bloodstream.

Beneficial stomach bacteria are also beneficial in strengthening the resilience of the digestive system and boosting immunity. Through this, unwanted materials from the intestines are prevented from leaking out, thus preventing inflammation and negative immune responses.

Apart from inflammation, not having a balanced set of gut microorganisms may make a person susceptible to metabolic syndrome, Type-2 diabetes, Alzheimer's, heart disease, depression, and colorectal cancer. Probiotics help to regain the balance of gut flora, thus correcting these diseases.

Probiotics and Digestive Health
Constant and prolonged use of antibiotics causes adverse digestive health effects. Doctors have discovered that those individuals who take antibiotics consistently over a long time tend to suffer from extended spells of diarrhea. In spite of the infection being cured, the person still suffers from repeated diarrhea. This is because antibiotics are known to kill the good bacteria that occur naturally in the stomach. When this happens, the balance shifts in favor of the bad bacteria, resulting in their increased growth.

There have been recent studies that have shown how effective probiotics are in the treatment of diarrhea resulting from overuse of antibiotics. One prevalent digestive disorder that is treatable through consumption of probiotics is IBS (irritable bowel syndrome). Other ailments that are also treatable include bloating and constipation.

In fact, probiotics are able to deal with even more serious ailments such as Crohn's disease and ulcerative colitis, which are both different forms of IBD. The digestive system is also protected from infections that generally cause ulcers and stomach cancer. Such infections are usually a result of attack of the stomach lining by Helicobacter pylori. Individuals suffering from digestive problems or weight problems must take the step of incorporating probiotics into their everyday diet.

Fast Fact: Even though probiotics was discovered in 1908, Probiotics were only finally named in 1965. It took scientists about 60 years to come up with a name for the living microorganisms that benefit humans in countless ways.

Probiotics and Weight Loss

In a study conducted by the School of Medicine in Washington University in 2006, it was found that obesity is somehow linked to microbes. This shows that people who are overweight have a problem with the number and diversity of good bacteria in their stomach. Another study conducted in 2009 by the Center for Genome Sciences in Washington University showed that obese people tend to have less diversity in gut bacteria.

The British Journal of Nutrition published a report about scientists from Japan who discovered that people who consume probiotics lose weight and are able to stay lean. The scientists believe that because of consumption of probiotics, the walls of the intestines are less likely to leak, thus preventing the chances of suffering from Type 2 diabetes, glucose intolerance, and obesity.

There are numerous studies that indicate the effectiveness of probiotics to prevent the absorption of dietary fat. Another suggestion is that probiotics enhance the excretion of greater amounts of fats via fecal matter. The conclusion scientists have made is that probiotics aid in the absorption of fewer calories into the digestive tract.

So how exactly does probiotics help a person lose weight?

1. Increasing Angiopoietin-like 4 levels

This is a protein located in the human genes. Research conducted by the Karolinska Instituet's Department of Microbiology in Sweden has shown that probiotics are able to increase the levels of Angiopoietin-like 4, thus lading to a reduction in the body's ability to store fats.

2. Releasing Glucagon-like peptide-1 (GLP-1)

GLP-1 is a hormone found in the gut. It helps in the regulation of appetite. A 2006 study conducted by the Arizona branch of the National Institute of Diabetes and Digestive and Kidney Diseases found that raising the levels of GLP-1 helped the body burn calories and fat. Research from scientists in the Maryland branch of the institute discovered in 2013 that probiotics helped raise the GLP-1 levels.

3. Reduced Inflammation

Research shows that being overweight leads to brain inflammation. Two distinct scientific reports released in 2014 and conducted by Brazilian and German researchers showed that probiotics are able to prevent obesity, boost immunity, and improve the functioning of the digestive system thus reducing inflammation.

There are numerous other benefits that probiotics offer the human body.

•Probiotics lessen the symptoms of psychological ailments such as clinical depression and anxiety, which are caused by brain inflammation. There is sufficient evidence of this benefit provided by two separate scientific publications by the Gut Microbes Journal (2011) and Current Opinion in Biotechnology (2015).

•Eating more probiotic-filled food helps improve the functioning of a person's immune system. This reduces the likelihood of contracting infections such as the common cold and vaginal infections. This was discovered in 2014 by Turkish researchers from Acibadem and Suleyman Demirel Universities. According to Britain's Journal of Nutrition published in the same year, US and UK scientists discovered that probiotics can effectively treat patients suffering from acute infections of the respiratory system.

•The Hypertension Journal published a study that revealed the positive role played by probiotics in the management of blood pressure and cholesterol. This surprised many because consuming more probiotics-rich foods had a similar effect to cutting down salt intake. This discovery further enhances the importance of probiotics.

•Studies conducted in Finland (2013) and the United States (2014) proved that adding probiotics to skin and make-up creams helps reduce skin disorders and allergies, including acne, rosacea, and eczema.

Are There Potential Side Effects?
It is important to always consult your physician before taking any dietary supplement. Though probiotics are safe, people who have excess bacterial growth in their bodies are not advised to take them. One example of an ailment that discourages consumption of probiotics is Small Intestinal Bacterial Overgrowth. Anyone with an immune system that is severely damaged, for example, due to HIV/AIDS, should not take probiotics.

Regular people may experience some digestive discomfort after a few days of starting a probiotics diet.

The next chapter covers some of the common food items that are rich in probiotics.

CHAPTER 4: FOOD GUIDE FOR A PROBIOTICS DIET

All set to begin your Probiotics Diet? The benefits of this diet will be maximized when these probiotics-rich food, supplements, and skin products are used.

Food Items
Fermented food contain natural probiotics, which makes them the most preferred source of beneficial bacteria. Though there are some foods that are artificially fortified, the bacteria they contain cannot be compared to those that are naturally fermented. When foods are processed during the manufacture of fortified probiotic products, the good bacteria usually die. This makes them less healthy.

There are variations in the levels of live bacteria in packed foods. Foods labeled as raw, lacto-fermented, or unpasteurized usually have greater levels of probiotics. Certain yoghurts are sealed in a way that indicates the presence of live cultures, or they are labeled as containing at least 100 million cultures in every gram. Frozen yoghurt usually contains a mere 10 million cultures in every gram.

When introducing probiotics into a diet, a person should include such food in every meal for at least three times every week. If the goal is to maintain good health and weight, it is important to consume them daily.

The list of food items below comprises the best sources of probiotics:

1. Raw Cheese
Opt for soft cheeses that are made from cow, goat or sheep's milk since they contain more probiotics. Always choose cheese that is raw or unpasteurized.

2. Yoghurt
This is the most popular probiotic-rich food. The best options are Greek yoghurt or those made from cow, goat, or sheep's milk. Always verify that the yoghurt you are buying comes from grass-fed livestock.

3. Kefir
This dairy product resembles yoghurt except it has a slight bitter and acidic taste. Kefir comes from Russia and Turkey, and is a mixture of kefir grains, yeast, and fermented milk. It has been consumed in these countries for millennia, and "kefir" in Russian actually means "feeling good." There are 10 – 34 different types of beneficial bacteria in kefir, with the large numbers being brought about by fermentation and yeast.

4. Coconut Kefir
This is a product of fermented kefir grains and coconut juice obtained from young coconuts. It is the non-dairy version of kefir made from milk, and has fewer beneficial bacteria. It still provides the required benefits, and tastes great when water, lime juice, and stevia are added.

5.Kvass
This is an Eastern European fermented drink that has been around for centuries. Initially, rye or barley was used during fermentation, but nowadays kvass is made from fermented beets, fruits, and root vegetables. It is slightly sour in taste.

6. Natto

This is a popular Japanese dish made from soy beans that have been fermented. It is high in probiotics content and provides health benefits such as boosting immunity, improving cardiovascular health, an aiding digestion of vitamin K2. Natto also contains the enzyme nattokinase, which is able to protect against cancer and inflammation.

7. Kombucha

This is Japanese black tea that is fermented with yeast. It has been part of the diet for over 2000 years.

8. Fermented Vegetables

Two perfect examples of fermented vegetables that contain live cultures are kimchi and sauerkraut, from Korea and Germany respectively. Sauerkraut is eaten in many different countries in Europe, though they are called a variety of names. In spite of the distance between the two countries, both dishes comprise fermented cabbages and are seasoned differently.

Sauerkraut is made from plain fermented cabbages, but kimchi is spicy and sometimes contains scallions and radish. They both contain high levels of enzymes and organic acids that aid in the breakdown of food during digestion. Furthermore, fermented vegetables make great side dishes that are healthy as well.

9.Human Milk

Using human milk as probiotics food is a bit controversial, even though it is an excellent source of good, live bacteria. The colostrum in mother's milk is what provides infants with their initial dose of antibodies and microorganisms that boost their immune system. Though it is broadly accepted to be a type of probiotics, some are not persuaded.

10. Natural Vinegar

This type of vinegar contains fermented rice, sugarcane, various fruits, coconut, and other diverse natural ingredients. They are similar to fermented vegetables since they too contain organic acids and enzymes that boost digestion.

Foods rich in probiotics can be either homemade or store-bought. It is cheaper, healthier and more hygienic to make them from scratch. The internet has numerous instructional resources on how to do this.

Fast Fact: Asian and European diets naturally contain probiotics, with fermented dishes like yoghurt and sauerkraut being perfect sources.

Supplements

Supplements are the most preferred form of probiotics for people who can't stomach probiotics food items or do not have time to make them. Supplements may not be comparable to fermented foods in terms of potency, but they are still effective. Overdosing on them is also difficult, thus making them safe.

They can be found in powder, pill, or liquid form. When buying them, always ensure that you choose supplements that contain lactobacilli and bifidobacteria, since these two strains have been studied the most.

Certain supplements may use labels like "mega probiotics," though they still provide the same health benefits as the rest. The difference is that they contain a more diverse group of bacteria. They are ideal when changing probiotics each month.

Skin Products

Probiotics products applied onto the skin are good options for women. Studies show that skin disorders can be treated using probiotics skin products, such as skin creams, gels, and makeup.

It is also believed that probiotics have properties that help slow down aging. Certain bacteria attach to keratin on the skin, thus reducing inflammation, preventing dryness, and healing the external layers.

It is not enough to just take probiotics supplements to keep the digestive system healthy. Exercise and proper dietary habits are also crucial. A lifestyle that is healthy and active, with adequate sleep and a diet filled with organic, whole foods will also play a key role in promoting stomach bacteria.

CONCLUSION

It is my hope that this book will help you establish better habits. Read the book as many times as you wish and put into practice the contents written here. It is not enough to just read and walk away unchanged. There are people who won't even manage to finish this book, yet because you have done so, you have proven that you are able to change your life.

THANKS FOR READING

We really hope you enjoyed this book. If you found this material helpful feel free to share it with friends. You can also help others find it by leaving a review where you purchased the book. Your feedback will help us continue to write books you love.

The Smart Reads library is growing by the day! Make sure and check out the other wonderful books in our catalog. We would love to hear which books are your favorite.

SMART READS ORIGINS

Smart Reads was born out of the desire to find the best information fast without having to wade through the sheer volume of fluff available online. Smart Reads combs through massive amounts of knowledge compiles the best into quick to read books on a variety of subjects.

We consider ourselves Smart Readers, not dummies. We know reading is smart. We're self taught. We like to learn a TON about a WIDE variety of topics. We have developed a love for books and we find intelligence attractive.

We found that each new topic we tried to learn about started with the challenge of finding the pieces of the puzzle that mattered most. It becomes a treasure hunt rather than an education.

Smart Reads wants to find the best of the best information for you. To condense it into a package that you can consume in an hour or less. So you can read more books about more topics in less time.

Visit:
www.smartreads.co/freebooks
to receive Smart Reads books for FREE

Check us out on Instagram:
www.instagram.com/smart_readers
@smart_readers

Don't forget your 2 FREE audiobooks.
Use this link www.audibletrial.com/Travis to claim your
2 FREE Books.

SMART READS ORIGINS

Smart Reads was born out of the desire to find the best information fast without having to wade through the sheer volume of fluff available online. Smart Reads combs through massive amounts of knowledge compiles the best into quick to read books on a variety of subjects.

We consider ourselves Smart Readers, not dummies. We know reading is smart. We're self taught. We like to learn a TON about a WIDE variety of topics. We have developed a love for books and we find intelligence attractive.

We found that each new topic we tried to learn about started with the challenge of finding the pieces of the puzzle that mattered most. It becomes a treasure hunt rather than an education.

Smart Reads wants to find the best of the best information for you. To condense it into a package that you can consume in an hour or less. So you can read more books about more topics in less time.

OUR MISSION

Smart Reads aims to accelerate the availability of useful information and will publish a high quality book on every major topic on amazon.

Smart Reads hopes to remove barriers to sharing by taking the copyright off everything we publish and donating it to the public domain. We hope other publishers and authors will follow our example.

Our goal is to donate $1,000,000 or more by 2020 to build over 2,000 schools by giving 5% of our net profit to Pencils of Promise.

We want to restore forests around the globe by planting a tree for every 10 physical books we sell and hope to plant over 100,000 trees by 2020.

Doesn't it feel good knowing that by educating yourself you are helping the world be a better place? We think so too...

Thanks for helping us help the world. You Smart Reader you...

Travis and the Smart Reads Team

WHY I STARTED SMART READS

Every time I wanted to learn about something new I'd have to buy 20 books on the topic and spend way too long sorting through them and reading them all until I arrived at the big picture. Until I had enough perspectives to know who was just guessing, who was uninformed and who had stumbled upon something remarkable.

I wished someone else could just go in and figure that out for me and tell me what matters. That's how smart reads was born. I want smart reads to be a company that does all that research up front. Sorts through all the content that is available on each topic and pulls out the most up to date complete understanding, then have people smarter than me package the best wisdom in an easy to understand way in the least amount of words possible.

For example, I got a new puppy so I wanted to learn about dog training. I bought 14 different books about dog training and by the time I got through the first 5 and finally started getting the big picture on the best way to train my puppy she had grown up into a dog.

Yeah she's well behaved. She doesn't poop in the house. I can get her to sit and come when I call. But what if someone else went in and read all those books for me, found the underlying themes and picked out the best information that would give me the big picture and get me right to the point. And I'd only have to read one book instead of 15.

That would be amazing. I would save time. And maybe my dog would be rolling over, cleaning up after my kids and doing the dishes by now. That my friend, is the reason I started smart reads. Because I wanted a company I can trust to deliver me the best information in an easy to understand way that I can digest in under an hour. Because dog training is one of many subjects I want to master.

The quicker I can learn a wide variety of topics the sooner that information can begin playing a role in shaping my future. And none of us knows how long that future will be. So why not do everything we can to make the best of it and consume a ton of knowledge. And I figured all the better if I can also make a positive difference in the world.

That's why we're also building schools, planting trees and challenging ideas about copyright's place in today's world. Because as a company we have to be doing everything we can to support the ecosystem that gives us all these beautiful places to read our books. Thanks for reading.

Travis

Customers Who Bought This Customers Who Bought This Book Also Bought

Eating Clean: Detox, Reduce Weight, Fight Inflammation and Reset Your Body.

How To Run: Beginner Running Program. Learn to Run. Running to Lose Weight. Runner Form. Fun Run.

How To Control Alcoholism: Proven Techniques to Stop Alcohol Abuse, Overcome Dependency, Break Addiction and Recover Your Life

The Powerful Benefits of Myrrh: Effective Myrrh Recipes For Healthy & Beauty, Oil Pulling Therapy, Creativity, Aromatherapy and Improving The Mind

Mint As Medicine: Discover The Powerful Healing Properties of Herb in Treating Headaches, Allergies, Asthma, Clarity and Peace of Mind

Self-Esteem Supercharger: Build Self Worth and Find Your Inner Confidence

Natural Ways of Boosting Testosterone: How to Bulk Up and Put Your Sex Drive in Overdrive

Beginner Gardening: Growing Vegetables and Ornamentals

Epsom Salt: Holistic Recipes for Beautiful Skin, Pain Relief and Relaxation